Nursing Tales
from the
`Hood and
Suburbia

A different kind of love story

Nursing Tales
from the
`Hood and
Suburbia

A different kind of love story

BENAY ELAINE ADAM, R.N.
AND
MARY ELIZABETH BURGESS, B.S., M.S.

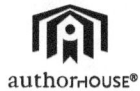

authorHOUSE®

AuthorHouse™ LLC
1663 Liberty Drive
Bloomington, IN 47403
www.authorhouse.com
Phone: 1-800-839-8640

Published by AuthorHouse   08/05/2014

ISBN: 978-1-4918-7407-3 (sc)
ISBN: 978-1-4918-7408-0 (e)

Library of Congress Control Number: 2014905198

In memory of Keith Burgess whose
wit and wisdom still inspire

Chap. 1

The woman was quite distraught. "You've got to save this cat," she said.

"But, ma'am, this is an ER."

"I know—emergency. That's why I brought him here."

"We only work on people, ma'am. This is a hospital for people. We don't treat animals." He said it really kindly.

She started to cry. Not just cry, but howl.

"I'm sorry about your cat," the doctor said.

She howled louder. "It's not my cat," she said. "I saw it get hit when I was driving down the street."

With that, the cat scratched her arm, jumped from her lap, fell on the floor and died.

She stopped howling. She looked at the black mass lying on her feet. "Well, see what you've done," she said.

"He's gone and died. Fine hospital this is." She flounced away, leaving the cat behind.

"Okay, doctor, now what?" Benay asked.

He picked up a black garbage bag used for biohazard waste, put the cat inside and deposited all in the trash container nearby.

"Takes care of one dead cat," he said.

"One black dead cat," Benay added.

CHAP. 2

This segment on *The News Hour* is interesting, but I get up to walk a minute as is my wont every half-hour to improve my back. This time to the kitchen to put my mug on the countertop, take two steps to my left to exit, catch my right shin on something, then defy all laws of physics and sail over the d-d-d door.

In mid-air I twist my body, the neurons saying Don't land on that ceramic floor, the one you recently installed to replace the soft vinyl: You'll smash your face or head.

Down I come, land on left ankle, feel and hear the sickening crack, the sickening stab of pain jolt me to my backside (but my hip is okay), half-way landing on the living room carpet, my legs under the dishwasher door. I'm facing back into the kitchen.

In the next second, you think, Some people navigate with a break so if someone helps on New Year's Day you'll still have your party, your 33rd year of serving kraut and sausage (in fact, you can still cut up the sausage—which you intended to start after The News Hour when you get back from the doctor's office. You do need medical attention.) Let's see, then you can call Helen; she'll be glad to help or maybe Debbie'll be in town. She said they might be. Who can you call to take you to the hospital, for in the final fracture of that second, the pain, the crack you heard, you realize it will require a hospital visit.

In the next second, you push the offending door up out of the offended way and—HELLO!—there's a foot, your foot, flopping ninety degrees to the outside.

This is a 9-1-1 deal, not a car deal.

For a few seconds you slide backwards diagonally across the living room carpet, pushing with your good leg (you hope it's your good leg) and your hands (they're intact, thank God), down the step into the sunroom and over to the swivel rocker.

The large, heavy ceramic blue-and-white garden seat blocks access to the phone which sits on a low stool behind it and beside the rocker.

O-kay. So, brilliant one, how are you going to get up on the chair? Only one way. You're going to do it.

So for an eternity you push upwards with hands and (you hope) that good leg, though the bad surely gets into the act too with the excruciation you feel.

You yell and yell at God to help you do this, to stop the pain long enough to do this, to give you strength-that's all you ask, all you'll ever ask—and on the fifth

4

try, She reaches down, pulls you up by the hair and lifts you like a feather onto the seat, the seat of safety, of help-within-reach.

When the attendants come, they shake their heads, staring. One says, "It's the tib. Where does it hurt?" and gingerly touches my ankle.

I hardly wince. "Here, below my knee it's sore."

He puzzles and touches.

"Wow. That's tender," I say. "Referred pain?"

"Probably."

Several hours later the X-ray technician says, "You have three breaks: spirals at the bottom of your tibia and fibula and a longitudinal below your knee, the top of the tibia."

"I knew it," I say half-triumphantly. "I told them it hurt there too."

"I didn't do her ankle," the tech tells the E. R. nurse.

When I get to my room, I realize God has already answered so many pleas, my quota surely has run out. The only one I pled after the number was dialed, was, since I knew I'd be at the mercy of many, was to have kind, compassionate, competent people, with my best interests in mind. The night nurse seems so, as did everyone in

E. R., even those who just came to gawk at my ninety-degreed foot.

By now it's after two a.m. Leaving that segment of *The News Hour* to, ostensibly, walk, has segmented me, and I try to get some sleep. It'll be a long day tomorrow, and maybe if I continue to be blessed, a long life ahead.

She's not my daughter. She's my stepdaughter, but I had nothing to do with raising her. She and her sister were already married when I married their dad.

She was here, when he died, not planned naturally, but she felt he might be worse than he let on. Her good nursing skills helped all three of us get through a very bad night and morning.

We cried, laughed, were amazed together: everything pretty much went the way he planned it—died in his own bed as we knew he wanted, even took his "toenails to the grave" just as he said he'd do when he refused the appointment I'd made with the podiatrist.

She returned many times, the longest visit for four months while she worked at our local hospital as a traveling ER nurse.

With her calm, cool manner (inherited from her dad) and laughter (inherited too from him), we got along fine. Took many trips together then and when, three other times, she worked sixty miles away and visited through the week. She prefers to work weekends, twelve hours three days, so when I went to that same local hospital last winter, having tripped over my dishwasher door that *someone* left down, she said, "I'm coming."

She found out about the accident before almost anyone else. Called me in the hospital that early Saturday a.m., before the surgery for my leg and ankle, wondering what happened.

"How did you know?" I asked.

"Your neighbor, the one who takes your paper to the door, saw the florist delivering the flowers I sent—" she always sends me flowers for my open house on New Year's Day, a late Christmas gift.

"He told the man you were in the hospital, and they called me to see if I should deliver them there."

"Gee, I guess not. Don't know how long I'll be in this room. They're talking like I'll have to go to a nursing home."

"Oh, no, you won't," she said. "I always told you if you ever needed me, I'd come. Unless you don't want me."

"Of course I want you. I just don't know when. I'll be in rehab for a while."

Many more phone calls ensued. And three trips to Lancaster. Four weeks of her life.

The day she walked into my room, the day after I'd started rehab, I could have cried. Now I'd have someone to bring mail, clothes from home. She could do my laundry too. She knew how to run my house. She just didn't know about the dryer.

Yet she became my angel, my savior.

CHAP. 3

"I'm going to tell you the first rule I learned in nursing: 'Kindness kills'."

She became Simon Legree, making me, a poor cripple, do everything for myself. First it was get my own breakfast. In a wheelchair with leg rests you have to keep lowering and raising to fit into the space under the table, get close to the refridge and sink, it ain't easy.

But somehow I manage to get the cranberry and almond cereal into the bowl, get the milk and orange juice, pour each into the proper containers, get my million-and-a-half pill bottles within reach. "Shall I fix yours too?" I ask with just a trace of sarcasm, knowing she usually has only coffee for breakfast, much, much coffee.

"No," she answers, ever so kindly. "I think I can manage."

She should. She gave us the coffee-maker for Christmas one year. My husband and I just looked at each other as neither one of us drank coffee. "It's for me," she said. "So I have coffee when I come."

"Your drug," he said. "Your addiction," I added.

But if it meant she kept coming, we were happy to have this otherwise unwanted appliance. Kept it under the sink until the day she arrived or for guests who were coffee drinkers.

"You're the perfect patient," she said.

I wanted to add, "Of course. I do everything myself."

But she said, "The people I treat in the E. R. back home, in the 'hood, expect everything to be done for them. And I do mean everything. Like go out and buy a morning paper when I'm trying to save someone's life. Like calling me an m-f-er when I don't."

"That's terrible."

"I tell them, black or white, 'Sir I'll talk to you and take care of you when you speak to me like a gentleman.' The women's language is just as bad."

"How do you tolerate it?"

"I don't know. The challenge I guess."

That's what's always driven her. She ran ambulance when she was in training, to earn money, but she loved the need to be creative in any emergency. Whether it was a fall from a ladder, a burn or drowning victim, a gunshot wound in the belly, quick thinking was the order of the day.

For four years she did ordinary bedside nursing, you know, take care of men after prostate surgery or vasectomies gone wrong, women after hysterectomies or breast surgery. Back rubs, daily baths, change of bedding, hooking up I.V.'s, pushing wheelchairs, requisitioning walkers, retrieving pills that roll out of reach of the patient, helping the patient make telephone calls from his bedside. All those little things that make nursing an exciting occupation.

Then an opportunity in the E. R. opened up. She applied, was accepted, decided to work the night weekend shift as her two kids could be looked after on weekends by their grandparents a block away. Weekends meant better pay. For thirty-six hours she got paid overtime, and holidays, double time.

After sixteen years at first Shelby, Ohio, then Manfield General, she traveled for five years to areas where ER nurses were in short supply. Then when she decided to settle down, she moved to Columbus to be near her kids, both adults by now. Ohio State University Hospital offered her salary and bonuses she couldn't refuse. Their satellits hospital was located in the ghetto, known to locals as The 'Hood. An advantage: it was not far from her apartment.

➢ ➣

Her goal of course in treating me so shabbily was to get me as independent as possible before she had to leave in seventeen days. I'd have gladly paid her to stay until I was fully rehabilitated, but she had to get back to tend to the house she bought the year before in a suburb of Columbus.

"Why are you doing this?" I asked at one point. "What did I do to deserve you?"

"You married my dad. Besides, he would want me to be doing this. And plenty of my co-workers take time off to go on mission trips to Central America. You're my mission trip."

It was a trip all right. She made God-knows-how-many trips back and forth to the hospital, to the grocery store, to the drug store, to K-Mart. She'd been at the house when the man came to measure for installation of a stair lift. He helped her make the house ready for me by taking doors off the upstairs bathroom, including the door between that and my bedroom so my walker would fit when I showered there, and the shower doors so I could get into the shower in the first place, once a special shower head with hose and bath seat were put in place. The doors they carried to the basement.

Dan also helped her carry the upstairs recliner down to the sunroom and carried that one up. Strong as an ox, she'd already moved at least a dozen pieces of furniture on her own, making room for a wheelchair and walker and hospital bed downstairs. That was needed as the stair lift wouldn't get installed till a week after I expected to be home. Dan also advised her to put stacks of dishes on the countertops where I could reach them from a wheelchair and to remove all throw and area rugs.

She planned meals and prepared them, except those brought in by friends until I got Meals-on-Wheels when she left. As mentioned, since she knew how to run the house (her dad would never let her empty the dishwasher, so she was proud to do that herself now), she took care of all my hospital clothes. I was expected to dress for therapy, so she brought in clothing I asked for.

We hacked one leg off the pants that wouldn't fit over my cast. She remembered to bring the scissors. When she bought her own meal to eat to share at meal-time, she shared part of her desserts with me. She brought my mail and checkbook, thought of stopping at AAA to get an application for a handicapped license, since most likely my car would be the one to be used for transport, it being large enough to get me and my clunk of a cast (later boot) into.

Our first morning together at my home I thanked her for something specific she'd done.

"Let's get this straight," she said. "One 'thank you' a day will be enough."

"Okay," I said reluctantly.

"Don't stomp on my joy," she said.

CHAP. 4

In the emergency room, things that happen are either bust-your-gut laughing or weep-your-eyes-out sad.

Sometimes people die. Despite the best efforts of doctors and nurses.

But sometimes people are hilarious. As in the case of the Cat Who Ended Up in the Garbage Bag.

One man, however, whose father was on life support and had become a vegetable, had to contend with other relatives who thought he should not be taken off the machine.

"You have no leg to stand on," one relative said. "He doesn't have a living will, and you're not his power-of-attorney."

It was true, but still the son was desperate. He told Benay his problem.

"Tell them," she advised, "that whoever makes the decision is responsible for his bills."

He brightened a little. He knew, of course, that he would be responsible. His greedy and guilty relatives would not contribute a penny. So he told them what she said.

After their brief confab, he said to Benay and the doctor, "Okay, take Dad off."

It was done. Benay was there when the man died. And when the son cried, she held his hand.

"You did the right thing. It's what he would have wanted."

"I know," he said. "Thank you. Thank you."

CHAP. 5

"Mary, what's wrong with your dryer?" she asked in alarm at the beginning of one hospital visit.

"Something wrong with it?" I answered coyly.

"I thought it was going to explode," she said. "I had to turn it off."

"It's got rocks in it," I said.

"That's sure what it sounds like."

"I'm sorry, I forgot to warn you about that. Last summer when I had pneumonia and the bad reaction to the antibiotic? I couldn't drive for so long, remember? Well, that's when it started clunking. I talked to several people about it, and they all said it was harmless. As long as it dried the clothes, they advised me not to replace it. I guess, since it was 22 years old, I should have replaced it once I started getting around on my own."

"Well, at least I know when I go back to the house, I can finish drying the clothes."

"Good thing. It's about time you bring me clean underwear."

"What's the matter? They starting to ban you from physical therapy?"

She bought me a journal to keep track of people to whom I'd want to send thank-you notes and an angel list to be called on after she left if needed.

"And also," she said, "to keep track of accomplishments."

So every day I wrote down, near the back, whatever new thing I did that day. At first it was, naturally, get my own breakfast. Then clean up after breakfast. Then it was navigate on the carpet without hurting my elbow pushing the wheelchair. Hop on the good leg lifting my weight on the walker without feeling I would topple over.

Sleep downstairs by myself. I insisted on this the third night. The first night Benay slept on the sofa across the room, getting up every time I got up to use the commode chair she'd placed beside my bed. "I'm fine," I said. The second night she woke when I peed five times that night.

"It isn't necessary for you to sleep down here," I said. "Please use the guest room. You'll get more sleep." I worried about her being on duty 24 hours.

She's a very deep sleeper as I'd found many times when I'd called her not knowing she'd finished a round in the ER. She didn't remember a word of the conversation. So we devised a plan. She put my cell phone on my bedside table and her phone on her bedside table—with the ringer turned extra loud.

The first time she slept upstairs was also the day I'd gone back to the surgeon to have the cast removed and a boot put on. "You can sleep in this or take it off, whichever suits you," he said.

I was used to the heavy cast and thought the boot, which was as heavy, reaching from toe to just below knee, would actually be comfortable in bed. It would be awkward and time-consuming to put it back on every time I went to the bathroom.

Wouldn't you know it, the first time I got up to use the potty chair, I lost my balance, stamped the foot down hard (the foot and leg I was to put no weight on for three months), and tipped over.

"Oh, God!" I yelled (as I'd yelled when I first fell over the dishwasher door). Again, she came to the rescue. This time I fell onto the potty chair, and it held my weight.

Before I'd barely got the words out, God (Benay) was down the stairs. (So she was sleeping lightly after all.)

"I'm fine," I said. "The chair caught me. Go back to bed."

After that, I truly believe she slept soundly every night.

With our various arrangements, she got adequate sleep. When she wasn't running errands, she took an afternoon nap along with me.

She worried about two things: that I'd become too dependent on the wheelchair and never get out of it, and that I'd not use the chair lift and sleep in my own bed.

The hospital bed with its electric control proved to be a boon. Because of damage to my upper body joints from receiving thirty electric shock treatments when I was twenty after the birth of my first child (the treatment for post-partum psychosis before lithium) I'd exacerbated these joints greatly, starting with tennis elbow in the hospital, from lifting my 115 pounds with every hop. With the electric aid of the bed, I didn't have to lift my weight from the bed every time I needed to get up.

The stair lift proved to be very useful when I needed to get a shower, which I finally did when the Occupational Therapist came to show me the safest way to do it.

This pleased both Benay and me, as, while I could bathe in a basin at the kitchen table (Benay filling the basin for me, one concession she made to my lack of independence), shampooing was another story.

Before I was able to go upstairs, we had to do it. "The O.T. in the hospital had me bend forwards over the sink in my room," I said.

"Hmmm," she said. She got the pink basin sent home from the hospital, the one I sponged bathed in at the kitchen table. "It's not deep enough," she said.

"Hmmm," I said.

She walked back to the kitchen. She appeared in the sunroom.

"Now hear me out," she said.

"Sure, Sweetheart, what's up?"

"We can use the lettuce drawer from the refrigerator."

"For my hair?"

"For your hair," the old authoritative voice returning.

"Hey, why not? I've got two of them. We'd just better not tell anyone who comes to my house that you drowned me in the lettuce drawer."

It worked perfectly well. It was deep enough, even had a slant that accommodated the angle I leaned from. In no time, my hair sparkled and glinted and I could stop scratching my scalp till it bled.

So I began a new page in the journal.

"Things that relieve stress." Number one on the list was: Lettuce drawer for shampoos.

One morning I woke up, very angry. Damn it, I broke my leg and ankle. I know it was my own damn fault, but damn it, the dishwasher door did it. I'm getting back at that damn door.

I told Benay my plan. "I'll kick it and let it know who's boss around here."

"But, Mary, you'll hurt your foot again."

"No, I won't. I'll kick it with the boot."

So after my bath, I told her I was ready, and while I took a healthy swing with the boot, she snapped a picture with her digital.

"*Das boot*, recorded for all posterity," I said triumphantly, and put the boot on.

Only thing is, with its hard metal tip, I'd dented the door.

"Well, I wanted to show it who was boss, didn't I?

"You sure did," Benay said.

I was philosophical about it though. "It's an indelible reminder of my tragedy," I said.

So the boot incident got added to my "stress" page.

On the "accomplishment" pages, the list had grown so considerably, I would have to jump out of an airplane without a parachute with two feet intact to top all the others.

Chap. 6

One day a woman came to the ER in agony.

"What's the matter?" Benay asked.

"I got the Blue Monster," she said, her face in a grimace.

"May I take a look? The doctor will want to know what the trouble is, and I have to document it on my report."

The woman pulled up her skirt. She spread her legs. Sure enough there was the smelliest, ugliest green-blue monster inside the woman's vagina.

"I see what you mean," my nurse step-daughter said, trying not to gag or hold her nose.

"Do something," the patient commanded.

"We will, ma'am, as soon as I get a swab and the doctor takes a look."

"Mercy me, is there no end to this?" the poor soul lamented.

"We hope to end it for you real soon," Benay soothed.

But, she says in telling this tale, *she* laments she'll never watch Sesame Street or Cookie Monster again.

Chap. 7

My greatest accomplishment, a stroke of genius, was turning on the garbage disposal without help.

About a week after we'd come home from the hospital, I decided I'd do the whole breakfast clean-up myself. Sometimes Benay didn't run the disposal as long as I liked (nor did anyone else who came in to take care of me), and I determined I'd not call her from upstairs nor wait till she came down.

I wheeled over to the kitchen sink, banana peel in my lap. It was obvious my arm was too short to reach the switch on the back wall. I needed an extension. I opened the utensil drawer. I got out a table knife. All it did was slip off the switch.

Hmm. I put the knife back. Next to it I spied the wooden spoons. I took out the longest one I could find, tried it, and the end slipped. I turned it around, and, *Voila!*, it worked. The bowl end was perfect to stay on the switch long enough to turn it on and off.

As I left it run long and loud, Benay came running down the stairs. "You did that?" she asked.

"Of course. Ain't I a genius?"

We were both proud of me. It deserved a red-letter place among all the other accomplishments, nearly twenty by now.

CHAP. 8

Camaraderie among ER workers is a lot like that among firemen and soldiers on the battlefield. When you go through crisis after crisis together doing your best, you forge very tight bonds.

Benay maintains friendships with several co-workers she met when she did her traveling. One she visits in Florida, another in North Carolina. My daughter is not only friendly and kind, she works hard. When she is not very busy with a patient, she helps other nurses who are.

When her dad went to the E. R. a few hours before he died, he was taken care of by a male R.N. Benay met when she worked at our local hospital. Between questions and hypodermics and waiting for the doctor to see test results, she and Jerry caught up a bit on old times. It was reassuring to know Keith was tended to by very caring persons those last few hours.

➤ ◄

Before Benay left the hospital after her first visit that January, she said she was going to have Robin make a bag for my walker to use when I got home. I discussed measurements with my physical therapist, and Benay and I discussed colors. She said Robin would use good judgment in choosing the fabric. She mostly did alterations and made other items, but Benay was confident she'd do a good job on the walker bag.

Did she ever! Not only was the pattern attractive, the fabric was sturdy, actually a scrap from upholstery work Robin had done. She had never made a walker bag before and charged Benay very little. Of course Benay paid more than the woman asked. I received many compliments on it, and when I wrote Robin a thank-you, I told her she should go into business. She was seriously considering it!

Near the end of Benay's stay with me, she learned that another co-worker, Helene, fell gravely ill. Helene was the oldest nurse in their department, in her sixties or early seventies, had loved nursing all her life. She had just nursed her husband through a very serious illness. She and Benay had become especially close partly because they often worked the same hours and on weekends. When her husband was ill, Benay often worked overtime to cover what would have been Helene's schedule.

She herself had lung problems and when she fell ill, she went into a coma. At a different hospital, she was put on life support, which only prolonged her life. After a considerable length of time, her husband and sons made the decision to stop the support.

The E. R. department rallied around the family. They were not poverty-stricken, but with the husband's long-standing illness, Helene's was the only income they had. So much money was collected, that an educational fund was set up in Helene's name to be given to a worthy nursing student.

I was impressed that when Benay asked for time off to be with me, the hospital gave her family leave, saying, as her stepmother, I was family. These days, with the nursing shortage, not all hospitals are that generous. She "paid" herself by using vacation and sick days, but the hospital saw that her hours were covered by other staff, and staff generously pitched in.

CHAP. 9

My step-daughter daughter wasn't always Simon Legree in caring for me.

As I lifted my 120 pounds on the walker and hopped on my good leg many times a day, my upper body joints broke down. They'd already been compromised by severe trauma when I was twenty and had given me problems for many years.

The surgeon was a "foot and ankle man"—now tattooed on his forehead—so he offered no help. Melissa, the physical therapist who came to the house, was, fortunately, also a massage therapist. She knew what to do to keep me exercising with the walker. Much of the time the pain would stop me after a few steps, so she'd massage my neck or upper back muscles to enable us to take a few more steps together. We'd continue like that for the rest of her hour or hour-and-a-half.

Early in that stage, I was getting my breakfast while Benay sat down for her coffee at the end of the table, our usual arrangement. I tried to lift and shake a nearly full orange juice carton and could not do it. I put my face in my hands and started to cry. "Damn it," I said in frustration, "I so wanted to take care of myself."

Benay took the carton and poured the juice. Her heart wasn't made of stone after all.

A day or so later, it was my wrists. Then my elbows. Then my hands.

When Melissa, my P.T., came a few days later, I told her Benay and I had thought up a new state lottery game.

"What's that?" she asked.

"It's called 'See Who Can Predict Which of Mary's Joints Will Give Out Next.'"

CHAP. 10

Before she became a traveling nurse, Benay and her two children lived in the house of an ER colleague, a gay man who went West for a year.

He came back for the holidays, as he had family in Mansfield, and escorted her to dinner more than once.

"It's safe," she said. She had no intention of re-marrying after two boyfriend situations that didn't work out well.

She had a heart for gays, and so when one partner ends up in the ER, she gives them a lecture about not just living wills, but wills in particular.

"You have no rights," she warns them. "No rights to make decisions, even to make visits in some circumstances, depending on other family members."

Who gets the death certificates, which next of kin are notified are but two of the complications that arise when the partnership is not legal. Of course, in most states, even the legal papers are not sufficient if there is no marriage license.

She has seen many very sad situations in which life-long partners are completely isolated at the time in both partners' lives when the other is most needed. She doesn't want to have to be witness to such heartbreak again. Ever.

CHAP. 11

MARY'S RULES FOR VISITING PATIENTS IN WHEELCHAIRS, I

1. Visitors should call first.

2. Visitors should make visits SHORT!

3. Visitors should come when they say they will and BE ON TIME.

4. Visitors should leave when they said they would.*

5. Visitors should adjust to the situation.

6. Visitors should help the patient adjust to the g.d. situation.

7. Visitors should not ask to ride the stair lift, not even dearly beloved grandchildren visitors.

8. Visitors should not use the word "ordeal" when describing what the patient has endured. They

may say, "What a terrible time you've had [and are having, they might add]," or "How awful!" or, better, "This was quite a challenge, wasn't it?"

9. Visitors should realize *they* will not have the courage, fortitude, energy, stamina or gutsiness to put up with such an ordeal, should they trip over a dishwasher door. (Which *somebody* left down. Benay says it was a gremlin.)

10. If visitors do not adhere to these rules, they may not be allowed in the door next time . . . . unless they have peanut butter crackers with them, a giant-sized box of p.b. crackers, not cheese p.b. crackers, gen-yoo-wine p.b.

*Or risk being booted out the door by the dreaded *Das Boot. Yah!*

CHAP. 12

Wherever Benay had gone as a traveling ER nurse, she was well-liked because she helped out other nurses when they were busy or had especially tricky patients' issues to deal with.

More than once, she caught grievous doctors' errors. Once it involved a patient almost receiving 100 cc's of a rescue-type medication instead of 10 cc's. She copied the order before it got faxed to pharmacy, and when the pharmacy questioned it too, the doctor, of course, corrected his order.

Another time she was about to insert a tube into a patient's left lung when some kind of intuition told her to re-check the X-ray again. Sure enough, the patient's heart was on the *right* side. In fact, he was one of those rare individuals who was born with all organs reversed.

(A few years later when my oldest step-granddaughter, Tracy, needed a heart catheterization, doctors found the same thing to be true for her!)

Each time Benay left a tour of duty, the ER staff threw a party: pulled pork or chicken done in a Crockpot for sandwiches; macaroni, potato, and seven-layer salads; assorted desserts—whatever a person's specialty was—and beverages.

Her first stint had been in Ashland, Ohio, home of her sister. Next came Tom's River, New Jersey. Then Lankenau Hospital (where her dad's heart by-pass surgery had been done) in Philadelphia. We saw a bit of each other when she was in Jersey, as it was about seventy miles from me. But she came very frequently when she was at Lankenau, only sixty miles away.

We went to Longwood Gardens and the Brandywine Museum in that area after I "helped" her move into a gorgeous upper-floor apartment on the Main Line. The building was old but had been well-taken care of and sported deep windowsills (for her many plants) and spic and span hardwood floors.

I slept in the living room on her comfortable couch and was wakened by birds chirping outside the window hiding somewhere in the many trees surrounding the building.

Since it was Spring, a feast for the senses greeted us from azaleas, rhododendrons, tulips, daffodils, and early day lilies every time we stepped outside the door.

Several times she came to Lancaster, usually Monday through Friday, as she worked Friday through Sunday from seven p.m. to seven a.m. We took day trips to art museums and other such cultural activities. It was a marvelous bonding time for us, preparing the way for even better times.

After Lankenau, Benay served at St. Joseph's Hospital in Lancaster, the same place where her dad had visited the ER umpteen times in the last three years of his life. From his heart by-pass in Philadelphia nine years earlier, tainted blood was hardening his liver with sclerosis. He showed no signs of hepatitis till our final trip abroad when we studied Impressionism in Paris and environs through an Elderhostel course.

After France we had traveled to Braunschweig, Germany, to meet with the first Friendship Force couple we had hosted 'way back in 1980. In the twelve intervening years we'd visited Ursula and Klaus in 1984, and in 1988 they returned for a month-long visit with their two teen-agers.

Although Keith had fallen ill in the very first week of this month-long trip abroad, he'd soldiered on to our final destination, Bruges, Belgium, "Venice of the North." We agreed it was the finest city of all in our review of our travels as he was going through the dying process the last three months of his life.

Benay had that same kind of determination as well as the same love of travel. In her various assignments she got acquainted with the area a day or two before she started to work, then on the days she wasn't visiting me, she toured the area. In upper New York state, sixty miles from the Canadian border, she fell in love with lighthouses after visiting Maine.

CHAP. 13

MARY'S RULES FOR VISITING PATIENTS IN
WHEELCHAIRS, II

1. Don't stay longer than a half-hour.

2. Don't ask to try it (the wheelchair) out.

3. Don't push the patient; he or she is perfectly capable of making it move by him—or herself.

4. Don't try to fiddle with the brakes. The patient may have had to have had them replaced several times and will not appreciate having to call a repairman one more time. He comes from a fur, fur piece, and said, next time, he will charge. A lot.

5. Don't bring ice cream. It takes too long for the patient to either put it in the freezer or dish it up. Since it would be impolite not to offer it to guests too, the patient could have difficulty handling several dishes. A tray is out of the question. Try

maneuvering a chair with a tray of several dishes of ice cream on it. I wish you luck.

6. Don't bring something hot, unless you want to re-heat it yourself. It is impossible for a wheelchair patient to manipulate hot things unless he or she stands up to reach the built-in microwave oven.

7. DO bring sweets. Chocolate. Chocolate with peanut butter. (Reese's giant-sized p.b. cups are most patients' preference. One person, herein unnamed, smears extra p.b. on top. Yummy.)

8. DO bring salty things: pretzels, p.b. crackers, cheese-filled cheese crackers (garlic cheese, please), chips of any type, Utz Grandma's (w/lard) chips preferred, but ANY sort of chip will do. Don't expect to be offered any of these. The patient will, in the interest of all humanity, wait till the guest leaves before indulging, esp. in p.b. crackers—unless the guest wants his or her hand broken.

9. DO leave in 15 minutes, unless you are going to the car to get more goodies. In which case, take your time.

10. PLEASE DO return, next time with a full-course dinner, to which you will be invited. Left-overs will, of course, be frozen for your next visit.

11. Thank you and PLEASE CALL AGAIN.

Chap. 14

After six years Benay and I still keep in touch. At times her health is not good—I worried about the nighttime coughing I could hear through the bedroom walls. Though she modified her caffeine addiction while she was with me, she never conquered the nicotine one.

My last visit was over Thanksgiving weekend in 2008 to see her remodeled house and to taste in person her famous brined turkey.

She looked like a scarecrow but was loathe to talk about her health, something of a fatalist like her dad. Her sister and I both worried when her tall frame continued to lose so much weight that her clothes hung on her. We all worried, knowing their mother had died of liver cancer.

Finally Brenda said, "Benay, you need to get tested if not for your own sake, for the kids." Steve lived at home permanently, and Andrea, a perpetual student, sporadically.

At last she reported over the phone she'd gotten tests, both for lung problems and colon problems. A breast lump was removed after her having to undergo the ordeal of two surgeries as she was "allergic" to the anesthesia. A colonoscopy had to be repeated as well, but polyps were removed successfully.

Shortly after her dad died, she slipped on the ice in the hospital parking lot and broke her wrist. It was the nastiest of breaks, necessitating a horrible external fixator, an outside rod screwed into bones, requiring several nerve blocks. Her picture appeared in the local newspaper with the surgeon who engineered the contraption.

I flew out for several days to tend to her, mostly in the emotional sense.

She worried she'd never work as an ER nurse as it was her dominant hand, and it had to be dexterous enough to give hypodermic shots. She missed three months of work with painful rehabilitation following the removal of the dreaded contraption that held her prisoner so long.

Now it's phone visits, she to check on me and my last remaining son, Scott. Me to check on Steve's health—he kicked an alcohol addiction when his mom came home permanently—as well as Andrea's progress in school and the latest boyfriend.

The bonds forged between us will hold forever. Once many, many years ago while her father was still living, she told me someone asked her what her relationship with her stepmother was like. "What do you call her?" the person asked.

She answered, "She's my friend."

As I told her the day she left me in February, 2008, to return to her family, we have a different kind of love story to tell. One forged out of mutual trust and respect. I think that's called LOVE in anyone's book.

ABOUT THE AUTHORS

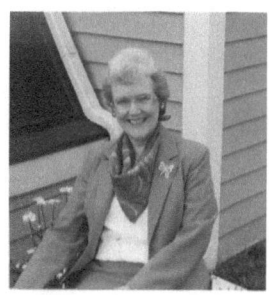 Retired reading and learning specialist, Mary Elizabeth Burgess won poetry prizes in 2009 and 2011 for "A Grocer's Picnic 1959" and "Grand Canyon Sunrise." Her short story, "The Flowerbed," won the WITF contest in January, 2013.

Ms. Burgess traveled extensively with her second husband, Keith, mostly to northeastern United States and Europe.They spent their honeymoon in wintry Russia in March-April, 1978, before The Wall fell. Mary and Keith studied under college professors Christian Art and Architecture in the U. S., as well as Impressionism in the Sorbonne in France.

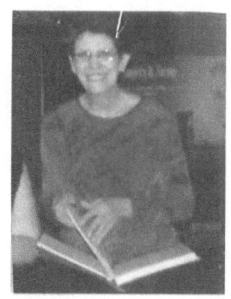 Benay Elaine Adam, with two children to raise after divorce, put herself through nursing school by "running ambulance," an exciting and challenging adventure. She became a traveling ER nurse for five years then was offered a job by Ohio State University hospital.

During much of that period she visited or lived with Mary. This cemented a friendship begun during the final illness of her father when, blessedly, she was visiting and helped her dad and Mary cope with a harrowing night of agonizing pain.

When asked once what she called her stepmom, Benay replied, "She's my friend."

www.ingramcontent.com/pod-product-compliance
Lightning Source LLC
Chambersburg PA
CBHW021040180526
45163CB00005B/2207